# Contents

# ABSTRACT

Moringa oleifera Lam. (Moringaceae) is a tree that is sometimes called the "Tree of Life" or "Miracle Tree." It is an economically important tree and vegetable, which has been variously used for treating different diseases. The leaves of the plant have been reported to have many pharmacological activities which include analgesic, antiinflammatory, antiasthmatic, antiulcer, antispasmodic, antibacterial, antihyperglycemia, antioxidant, anticancer, and larvicidal activities [64–67]. Toxicological studies on Moringa oleifera have shown absence of severe hepatotoxicity and organ damage except in very high doses. The acute lethality (LD50) test

3

of Moringa oleifera has been found to be relatively safe with the subchronic

toxicity studies, eliciting no significant difference in sperm quality, hematological and biochemical parameters in the treated rats compared to the control. Moringa oleifera has recently been reported to possess potent anticancer effects and exhibited synergistic effects with cisplatin. These and its longtime use in ethnomedicine have shown Moringa oleifera to be a good candidate for clinical trial studies.

# WHAT IS MORINGA

Moringa oleifera is a small, graceful, deciduous tree with sparse foliage, often resembling a leguminous species at a distance, especially when in flower, but immediately recognized when in fruit. The tree grows to 8 m high if allowed to grow without trimming. The bark of the tree is smooth, dark grey. The wood is soft. Leaves alternate, the old ones soon falling off. Leaflets are dark green above and pale on the under surface; variable in size and shape, but often rounded -elliptic, seldom as much as 2.5 cm long.

Almost every part of the plant is nutritious. In India, the pod is cooked as vegetable and sometimes exported to some countries for Indian expatriates. The root are definitely very good as substitute for horseradish. The dried and grinded leaf powder can be added to any kind of meal as nutritional supplement. The seed can be roasted and eaten.

# THE ORIGIN OF MORINGA

Moringa is said to have originated from India. As early as 2000 years BC, Moringa has been described as a medicinal herb in India.

In the annals of Ayurvedic Medicine, one of the oldest healthcare systems in the world, Moringa has been mentioned as a cure for over 300 diseases. Over the centuries, the Moringa tree has been carried to all the tropical parts of the world, where it readily takes root. Moringa tree is commonly used for food, for medicinal purposes, as a wind-break in fields, and many other purposes. Ancient Egyptians treasured Moringa oil as protection for their skin from the ravages of desert weather. Later, the Greeks found many healthful uses for Moringa and introduced it to the Romans. The moringa tree grows widely in Africa where up until recently it is used solely around houses to form hedges or to give shade.

# WHY MORINGA IS CALLED THE MIRACLE TREE

Many plants and trees are beneficial to mankind, but few are as giving as the Moringa Oleifera tree. Moringa trees have a list of medicinal, nutritive, and practical uses that are second to none. A single Moringa tree can provide leaf for nutrition, oil for cooking and healthy skin, seed cake for water purification and wood to build shelter and keep you warm. The Moringa tree thrives in arid conditions, where its benefits are most valuable and most needed. Living up to its nickname as a miracle tree, Moringa is the basis of many health and nutrition programs funded by various charitable organizations. Moringa leaf capsules and bulk leaf powder are an incredible nutritional supplement with more than 30%

protein, all of the essential amino acids, 27 vitamins and 46 antioxidants. Moringa is truly a gift to the impoverished in parts of the world where life is hard and nutrition is scarce.

In many cultures, the phrase used to identify the Moringa tree translates as the Tree of Life. This term may bring religious meaning to mind, but in truth, cultures worldwide share the symbolism of the Tree of Life as a symbol for life, growth and change. Moringa is known as a tree of life because its many gifts are life-giving. Amazingly, in addition to basic nutrition and water-purifying properties. Moringa's health benefits have been used in the prevention/management of more than 300 ailments. Within the past ten years, Moringa oleifera, a tropical, multipurpose tree has grown from being practically unknown, even unheard of, to being a new and promising nutritional and economic resource for developing countries. The leaves, which are easy to grow and rich in proteins, vitamins and minerals, are becoming widely used in projects fighting against malnutrition. Producing moringa leaves is also a means of generating agricultural income, developing the food processing industry and founding new businesses.

## MORINGA, A GREEN "SUPERFOOD"

The leaves of Moringa, this small tree found in the tropics, were recently identified by the World Vegetable Center (Taiwan) as the vegetable with the highest nutritional value among 120 types of food species studied. Easy to cultivate and resistant to drought, this tree produces abundant leaves with a high concentration of proteins, vitamins, and minerals: 100 grams of fresh Moringa leaves provide the same amount of protein as an egg, more iron than a steak, as much Vitamin C as an orange, and as much calcium as a glass of milk. Moringa grows throughout the developing world and has already been used by programs to reduce child malnutrition in India. For over forty years, WORLD HEALTH ORGANISATION (WHO) has been using the tree to combat malnutrition. Its dried leaves, in powder form, can be easily preserved and used. Eating 30 grams a day, a child can satisfy all his daily requirement of Vitamin A, 80% of daily calcium needs, 60% of daily iron needs, and nearly 40% of protein needs.

Given the world food crisis, the use of local resources like Moringa is critical to reduce the dependence of developing countries n imported goods, and to improve nutrition among poor households. Two or three trees in a courtyard are sufficient for the needs of one family.

# BRIEF AMAZING FACT ABOUT MORINGA TREE

Below are some amazing facts about this miracle tree.

Medicinal Values of Moringa starting with the Leaves:

Nutritional analyses indicate that Moringa leaves contain a wealth of essential, disease-preventing nutrients. They even contain all of the essential amino acids, which is unusual for a plant source. Since the dried leaves are concentrated, they contain higher amounts of many of these nutrients, except vitamin C. According to Producer and Philanthropic organization Kuli Kuli, Gram for gram, the Moringa leaf contains:

1. two times the amount of protein of yogurt

2. four times the amount of vitamin A as carrots

3. three times the amount of potassium as bananas

4. four times the amount of calcium as cows' milk

5. seven times the amount of vitamin C as oranges

Vitamins & Minerals-

Moringa is a very rare plant in that it contains much of the vitamin and mineral spectrum in including: Vitamin A, B, C E, calcium, magnesium, phosphorus, potassium, zinc and more.


Protein & Amino Acids-

Dried Moringa Leaves contain not only a respectively large amount of protein for a leafy green, but also, all the essential amino acids. This in combination with the vitamin and mineral spectrum creates a very well rounded, and as we shall discuss, beneficial nutrition source.

Moringa Leaves relieve headaches, expel worms, relieves swelling, and heals skin diseases, inflammation of the eyes and ears, bronchitis and inflammation of mucous membranes, scurvy and increase milk production (quality and quantity) in lactating women, i.e. breastfeeding mothers.

Moringa Flowers

Moringa flowers are a good tonic, expel worms, treat tumors and enlarged spleen, relieve sore throat, and treat anxiety. The flower juice generally improves the flow and quality of the milk of a breastfeeding mother. It also encourages urination and fight against urinary problems. As a cold remedy, drinking of tea made from moringa flowers are very helpful.

Moringa Pods & seeds

They purify water, treat tooth ache from tooth decay, expel worms, treat problems of the liver and spleen, and relieve joint pain. The pods play a vital role in treating diarrhea and malnutrition. The seed can be used as a special relaxant for common epilepsy. The seed also aid sleeping after a very stressful day.

Moringa seeds are highly effective against Pseudomonas aeruginosa and skin-infecting Staphylococcus aureus (bacteria). The also contain fungicide terygospermin and potent antibiotic.

Moringa Roots

The roots are used as a laxative and to treat spasms of the colon, treat circulation problems, high blood pressure, kidney dysfunctions and low back pain; for gout, asthma and hiccoughs.

The bark and roots are used for circulatory and cardiac problems, for inflammation and as a tonic. The bark is truly digestive and an appetizer as well.

In India and Senegal, roots are nicely pounded and properly mixed with normal salt for making a poultice for the treatment of articular and rheumatism pains. This type of poultice is also used for relieving kidney or lower back pain in Senegal. The nerve paralysant (alkaloid spirachin) has been found in its roots.The gum is abortifacient, astringent and diuretic, which is used against a common problem, asthma.

Other views

Fresh leaves are said to be inserted into the nose of a comatose person, who is then aroused from the coma!

In laboratory tests the leaf extract of Moringa lowers blood sugar within three hours, heals stomach ulcers, is a powerful muscle relaxant, reducing blood pressure and causing sleep. Also in laboratory tests, juice extract from leaves and bark have shown antibacterial and antiviral properties, and show strong activity against the tuberculosis bacteria.

HOW TO EAT MORINGA SEED TO ACHIEVE DESIRED RESULTS

Below are few tips to help you make the most of the moringa seeds you've got so as not to do more harm than good to yourself. Did I say "more harm"? Yes! Too much of everything is BAD!

1. DO NOT EAT MORINGA SEEDS ON AN EMPTY STOMACH!

It is not medically good to eat moringa seeds when you have not taken any food before, especially early in the morning. What will happen if I do that? Good question. It may cause you to purge. Although that is not a bad one entirely because it is the after -effect of detoxification. So if you are ready to frequent the toilet, go ahead... But I will advice you to do that only when you want to see that result-DETOXIFICATION.

## 2. DO NOT EAT MORINGA SEEDS WITH THE COVERING (PEELS)

It is not hygienic eating the moringa seeds with the bark on. Again, for every rule there is an exception. Therefore for those who want to achieve faster weight-loss, make sure you wash the moringa seeds with water and salt and rinse at least twice.

DON'T USE ANY DETERGENT FOR WASHING! Laughs...


## 3. DO NOT EAT MORINGA SEEDS IF YOU ARE PREGNANT!

Now read this slowly again and again... If you are pregnant, please STOP taking moringa seeds until after delivery. But can you be taking other moringa products, Yes! Especially the moringa leaves/leaf powder. But for the seeds, please STOP! Incidentally, if you are looking for the fruit of the womb, or trying to conceive (TTC), moringa seeds are A MUST for you. Can you see the irony there? Yes, that is MORINGA for you.

## 4. DO NOT EAT MORE THAN TWO (2) MORINGA SEEDS PER TIME!

Yes! You read right. Eat a maximum of two (2) moringa seeds per time. In fact, if you are eating for the first time, start with one (1). Subsequently you may take two. How many should I take in a day? Did I hear you ask that? Four*. Why did I asterisk the four? Because that is the very much we recommend to our clients, depending on their peculiar condition.

## PREPARING MORINGA LEAVES FOR DRINKING

Moringa teas are available in grocery stores, but some people prefer to make it themself, so far you have access to Moringa tree. The process is definitely simple, although harvesting the leaves from the stem can be time-consuming.

When making tea, you may either steep the fresh Moringa leaves in hot water or dry them up so you can use them for later when you're recreating different Moringa tea recipes.

Method 1: Make dry leaves

1. Prepare your moringa oleifera leaves (select mature ones, not young). There is no need to collect flowers or seeds if you only wish to make tea from the leaves of

this plant. If you can gather 3-5 stalks, it will be more than enough.

2. It is necessary to dry all the leaves beforehand. Therefore, place fresh leaves on a flat surface and let them air dry. Sometimes it takes a day, and sometimes it can take a couple of days or even 1-2 weeks. You will know that your leaves are ready to be used for making tea when they become crisp.

Tips: users who have a special food dehydrator can dry their leaves in a couple of hours.

3. Separate dry leaves from stalks if you want to. Some Nigerians love adding parts of the stalk into their tea along with moringa leaves because they contain fiber.

4. Place your leaves with or without stalks (it's up to you) into a blender or grind them in a different way (for example, you can try using your coffee maker). You

should turn all the dry leaves into small pieces. But don't grind for more than 30 seconds or they'll become powder instead of pieces.

5. If you have some tea bags, you can add the blended moringa leaves into the bags and store them like this. If you have no bags, use a glass jar for this purpose. It is better to keep your product in a dry place. This way it will last longer.

6. Since we are talking about how to make moringa tea, let us learn what you can do with the product you have prepared. Boil some water. Take a cup. Add a teaspoon of moringa leaves into the cup and pour in hot water just like you do while preparing regular tea. You can add some sugar or honey based on your taste. It is also to add fresh lemon juice into your tea. It will taste

incredible and offer you many useful elements and vitamin C.

Method 2: Use fresh leaves

It is also possible to drink tea made from fresh moringa leaves, which you do not dry beforehand. If you are a fan of such method of cooking this product, here is a short guide for making your useful beverage:

1. Gather 0.5 cup or 1 cup of fresh moringa leaves. Do not use stalks, simply separate the leaves with your hands.

2. Take a deep pot and add 3 cups of water. Put it on a stove and turn on the fire.

3. Add fresh leaves into the pot and boil moringa leaves for approximately 5 minutes.

4. Let the beverage cool down.

5. Pour your freshly cooked moringa tea into a cup, add sugar to your taste or replace it with a teaspoonful of honey, and drink it this way.

BENEFITS OF MORINGA

1. Lower Blood Pressure

Moringa works perfectly to lower blood pressure. The obesity level in the Western world is more rampant which also makes high blood pressure become more and more of an issue. High pressure can cause serious cardiovascular issues such as heart attacks and strokes.

To naturally lower blood pressures, it is suggested you take part in exercise regularly and lead a healthy lifestyle. However for some people whom are already at a dangerous stage, exercise may be out of the question, so medication will be the only alternative.

Research show that Moringa and its seeds can lower blood pressure; however more research is still being done to confirm these theories fully. The current results prove Moringa seeds reduce oxidized lipids and safeguards heart tissues from constructional damage. Consult your doctor before trying Moringa seeds as a blood pressure balance.

Each part of the Moringa Plant has its own benefits. Whether you're using the leaves, flowers, roots or seeds, each will aid the body in a number of different ways.

2. Diabetes – blood Sugar Levels

Alongside its ability to lower blood pressure, this goes hand in hand with the seed's ability to lower blood sugar levels.

The seed's rich zinc concentrate helps to regulate the secretion of insulin.

As this becomes more normal, the blood sugar levels also become regular. Although studies have only been done on lab rats so far, this discovery could lead to preventative and therapeutic management of diseases such as diabetes

3. Cholesterol

With zero presence of cholesterol in the seeds, Moringa is known to reverse the effects of high cholesterol. High cholesterol rates in the blood are linked to the development of heart disease. In Ancient Thai medicines, Moringa is classed as a cardiotonic which controls and improves the way the heart contracts.

Moringa products monosaturated fatty acids called oleic acid. Oliec acid (often found in olive oil) has many benefits for our health and can prevent blood clots or cardiovascular diseases. If you're looking to improve your diet, aim to replace saturated animal fats with Moringa to keep your cholesterol levels down.


4. Beautiful Skin

Oils are extracted from the seeds to create a number of cosmetic products. The oils contain up to 30 antioxidants and a surplus of Vitamin A which are the ideal choice for skin products.

Vitamin A enhances the firmness of the skin to appear more youthful and fights against signs of aging and stress. This is done by promoting collagen formation within the skin cells.

The fatty oils are known as Ben oil and it forms roughly 40% of the seed. It has no smell or colour and tastes sweet. The skin absorbs the oils without saturating the oils on the surface of the skin – and receives all the nourishing qualities the oil has to offer. The oil works as both a moisturizer and an antiseptic cleanser to get rid of acne, pimples and blackheads.

To use on the face, all you have to do is apply a few drops to the skin and massage it in like any other moisturiser or massage oil.

5. Moringa Seeds and Weight Loss

Ben oil from the seed extract breaks down saturated animal fats in the diet and works with the digestive system to get rid of the fats we don't need. By doing this, the oil reduces belly fat.

## 6. Anti-Inflammatory

The Moringa plant is well-known as a natural anti-inflammatory, so the seeds are no different. Moringa seeds can reduce soreness and boost the health of our joints. Strengthening the joints with amino-acids and proteins enables sufferers of arthritis and other disorders to live a more independent life.

## 7. Immune System

We're all aware of the amazing benefits of Vitamin C. Moringa seeds host home to a huge level of Vitamin C which makes them ideal for boosting the immune system. The vitamins work to fight against free radicals and infectious agents.

The huge amounts of nutrients digested from eating the seeds of the Moringa plant boost the immune system and help to heal bruises, cuts, burns and minor injuries in a more timely manner.

8. Teeth and Bones

Rich in Zinc, Calcium and plenty other minerals, Moringa seeds ensure overall well-being.  Other minerals found in the seeds such as Iron reduce and prevent anaemia symptoms. The calcium keeps bones and teeth strong. Zinc has been known to facilitate in spermatogenesis (the process of sperm production in men).

9. Water Treatment

On a more charitable scale, Moringa seeds, oil and seed cake are being tested and used for treating dirty water. This paves the way to cleaner drinking water facilities in third world countries and could fight against life endangering diseases in these areas.

There's plenty more Moringa seed benefits too, like helping with weight loss, constipation or insomnia.


10. Moring Seeds Encourage Hair Growth

By looking after our bodies internally, Moringa seeds can benefit our hair. The vitamins A and C contained in the moringa seed are good for making your hair stronger and growing faster. Having healthy hair is great for both women and men. The natural herbs work great on helping the hair cells to repair and feeding your follicles with 'food' (nutrients) they require. Vitamin C present in the seeds can encourage and improve blood circulation through the scalp to help hair follicles grow and strengthen. This results in fully, healthier hair.

Zinc and Vitamin A also promote hair growth. Nourishing the hair tissues and repairing the cells, Zinc keeps sebaceous glands unclogged so the follicles can absorb as much nutrients as possible.

Not only are the seeds great, but the oils extracted from the seeds can be used as shampoo – to help get rid of itchy scalps and dandruff.

With these striking results, it's no surprise how the Moringa seed has become a well-known super food across the globe. These crucial vitamins are essential for the body to fight free radicals and prevent severe oxidative damage.

11. Help with constipation or better digestion

The plant contains fiber that can improve your digestion and is another health benefit of moringa seed. It is a great way to boost food moving in your system. Fiber wouldn't hurt, this is for sure.

12. Aids in sleeplessness – insomnia.

Moringa leaves improve sleep. The factor contributing to this is the amino acid tryptophan. It is important in the production of the neurotransmitter serotonin and the hormone melatonin, which regulates the sleep cycle. The leaves also contain vitamin B6 - another necessary player in the production of serotonin.